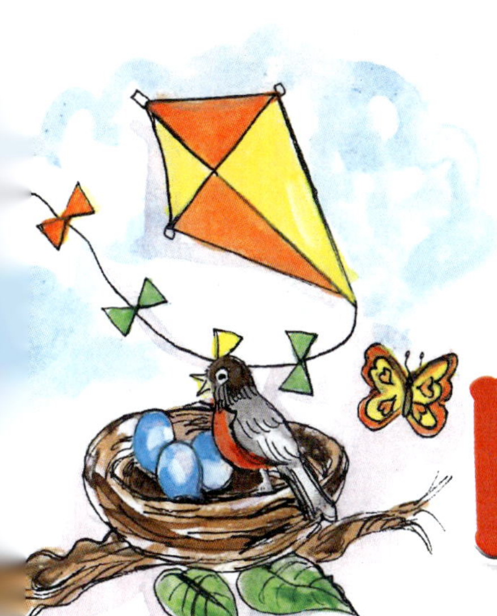

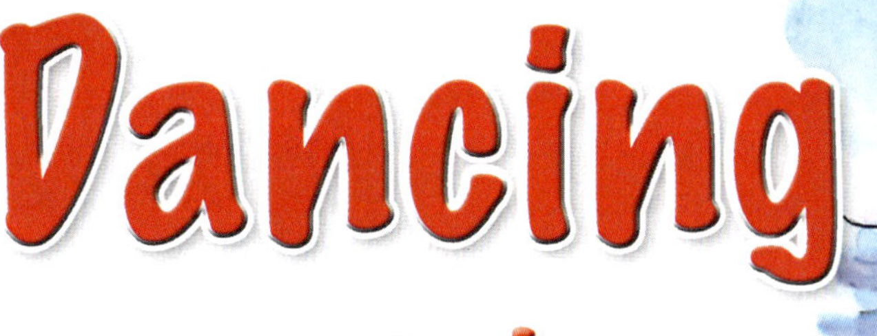

Dancing with Great Grandma

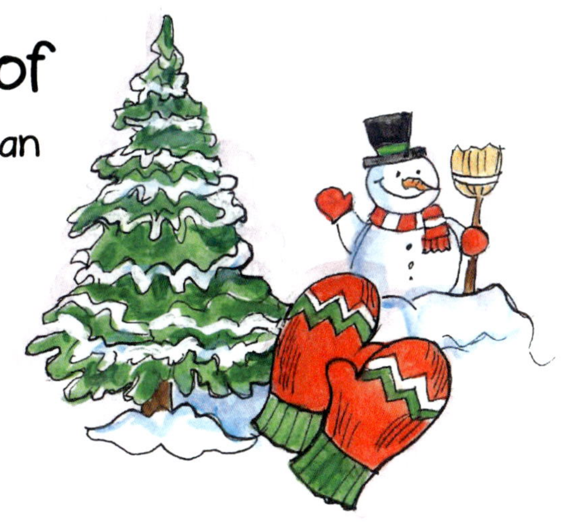

By Rose Klopf Tithof

Illustrated by Carilyn Teichman

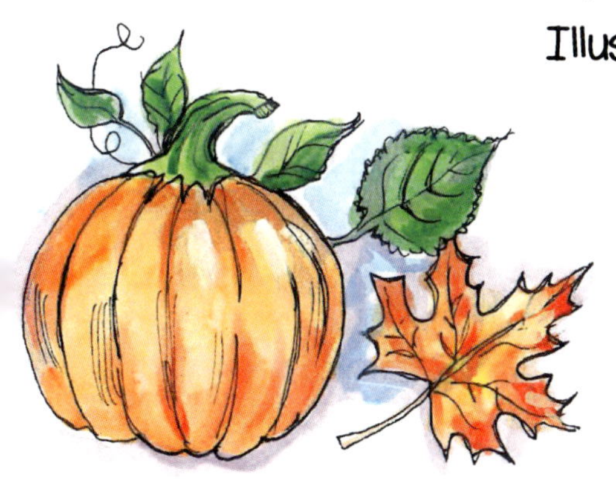

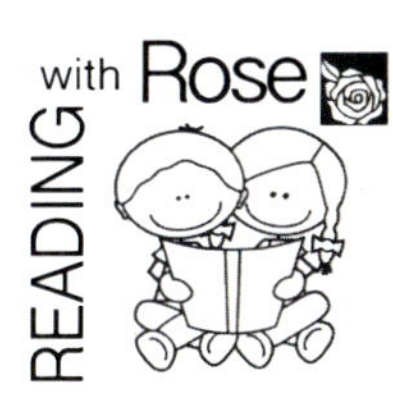

ISBN 978-0-9891006-8-7
Published by Reading with Rose

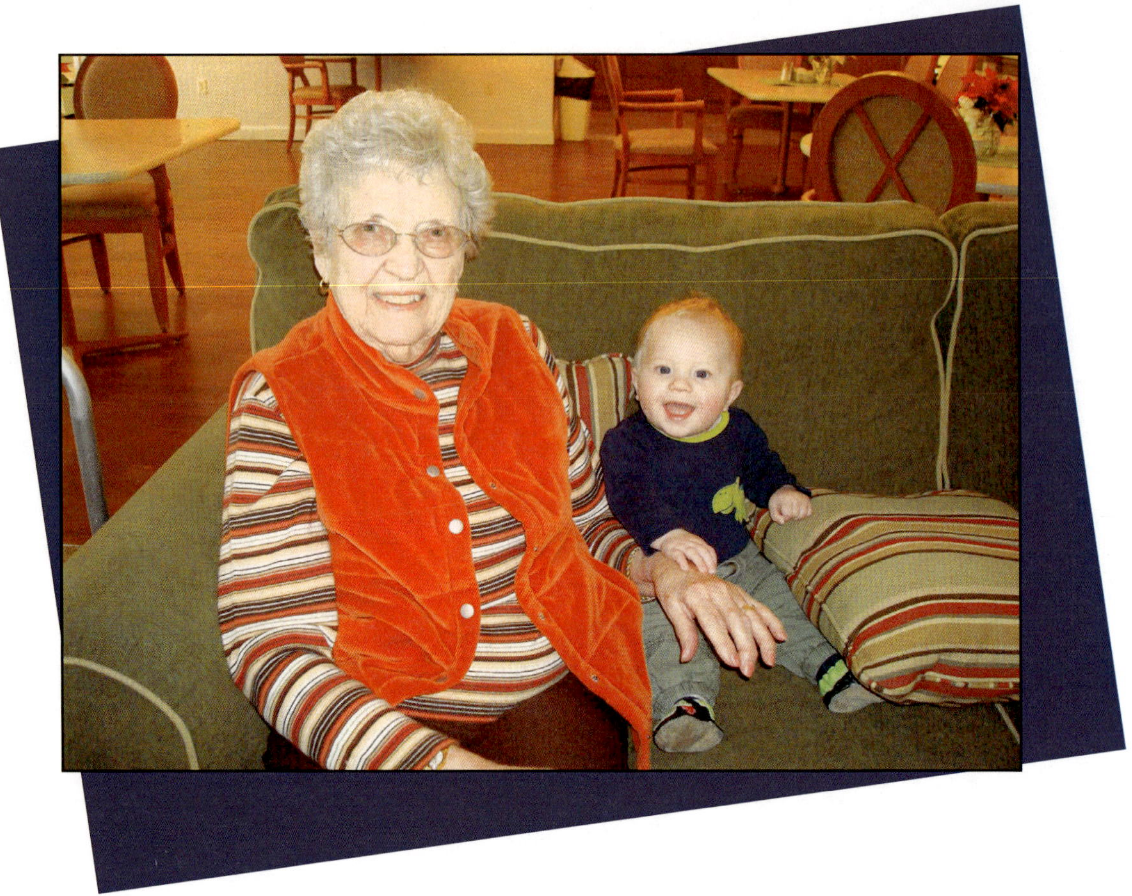

This book is dedicated to the two main characters—my mother, Lillian Bothe Klopf (Great Grandma), and my grandson, Lawrence Danek (Law), who easily “dances” into the hearts of those he meets.

Special thanks to Union Court Assisted Living, St. Charles, Michigan for the love and care they demonstrated during my mother's stay in their facility and for all of the "fun" activities that they scheduled.

Additional thanks to Paul and Lee Danek for the photos they took, which have now become the painted illustrations done by my very talented illustrator, Carilyn Teichman.

Thanks also to Dave Rusz, the pianist who still faithfully plays beautiful music every Wednesday at Union Court.

Thanks to Fred Arndt for the use of assorted Christmas ornament images from his collection.

I could not have completed this project without the help of Julie Wenzlick. Not only is she an excellent editor, she is able to prepare the text and illustrations for publication.

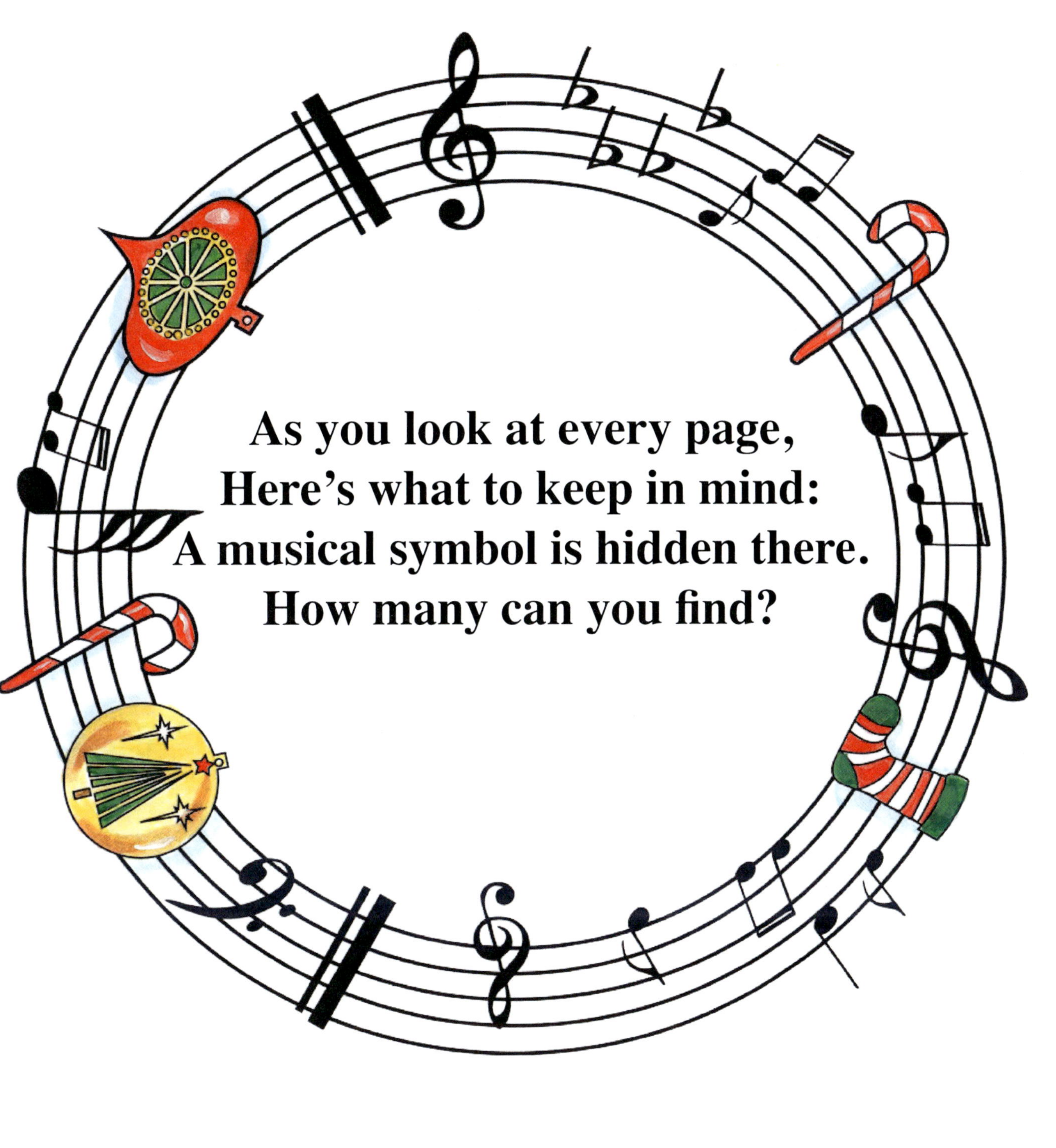

As you look at every page,
Here’s what to keep in mind:
A musical symbol is hidden there.
How many can you find?

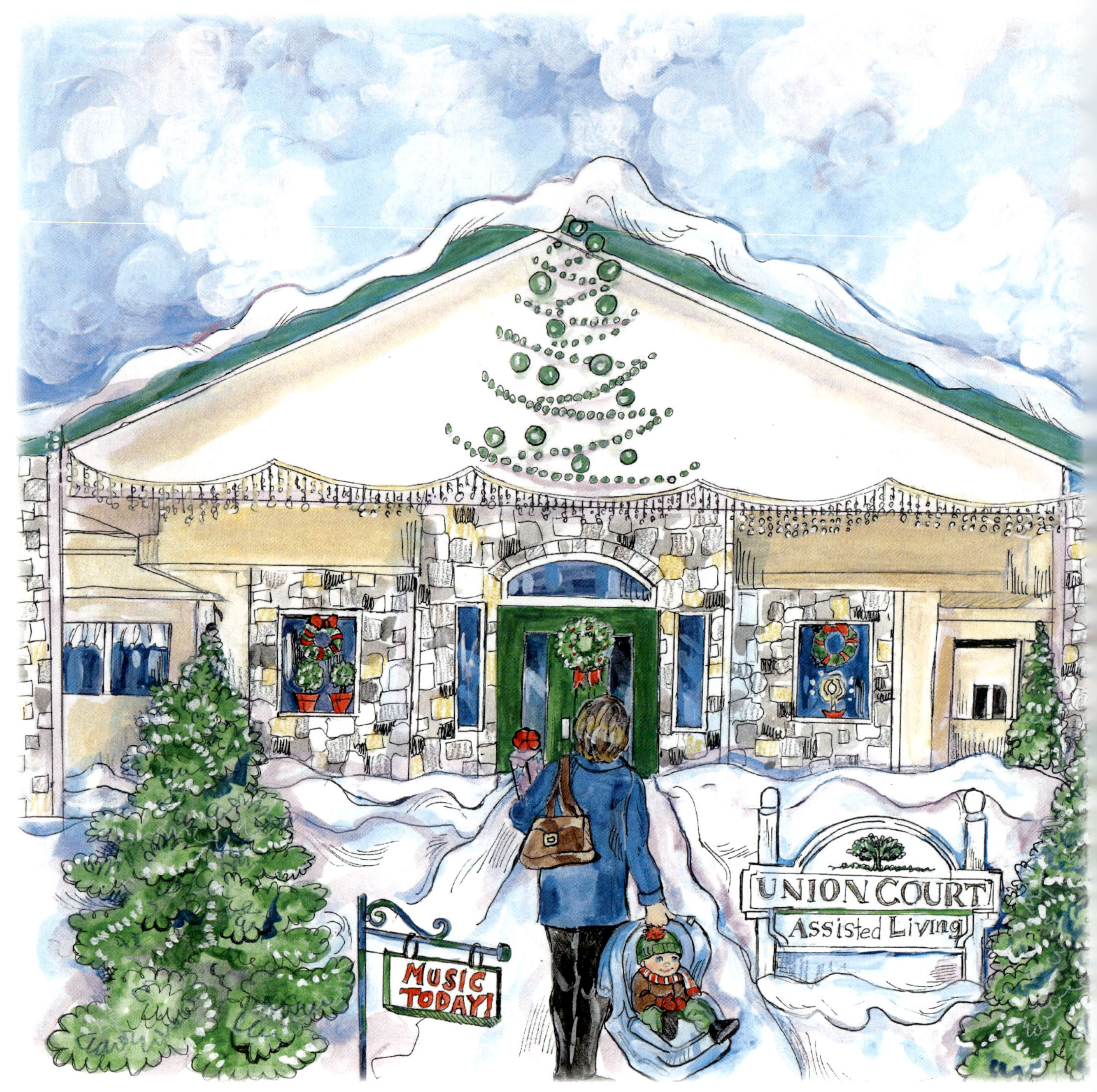

Great Grandma Lillian lived in an assisted living home. Her daughter, MiMi, often visited her mother with great grandson, Law. They especially enjoyed musical Wednesdays.

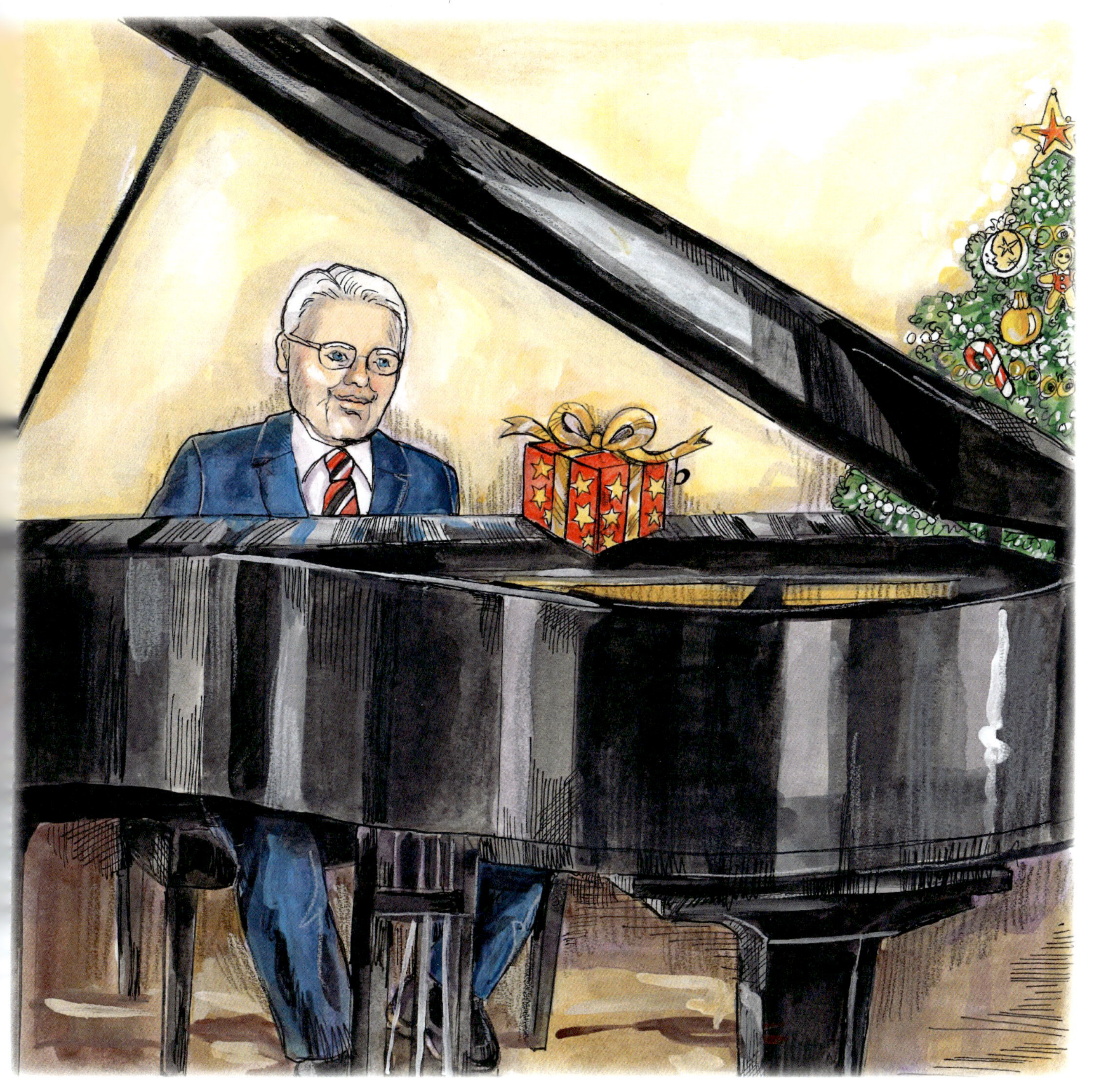

Each week, Dave came to play for these elderly folks because he knew the music brought them great pleasure.

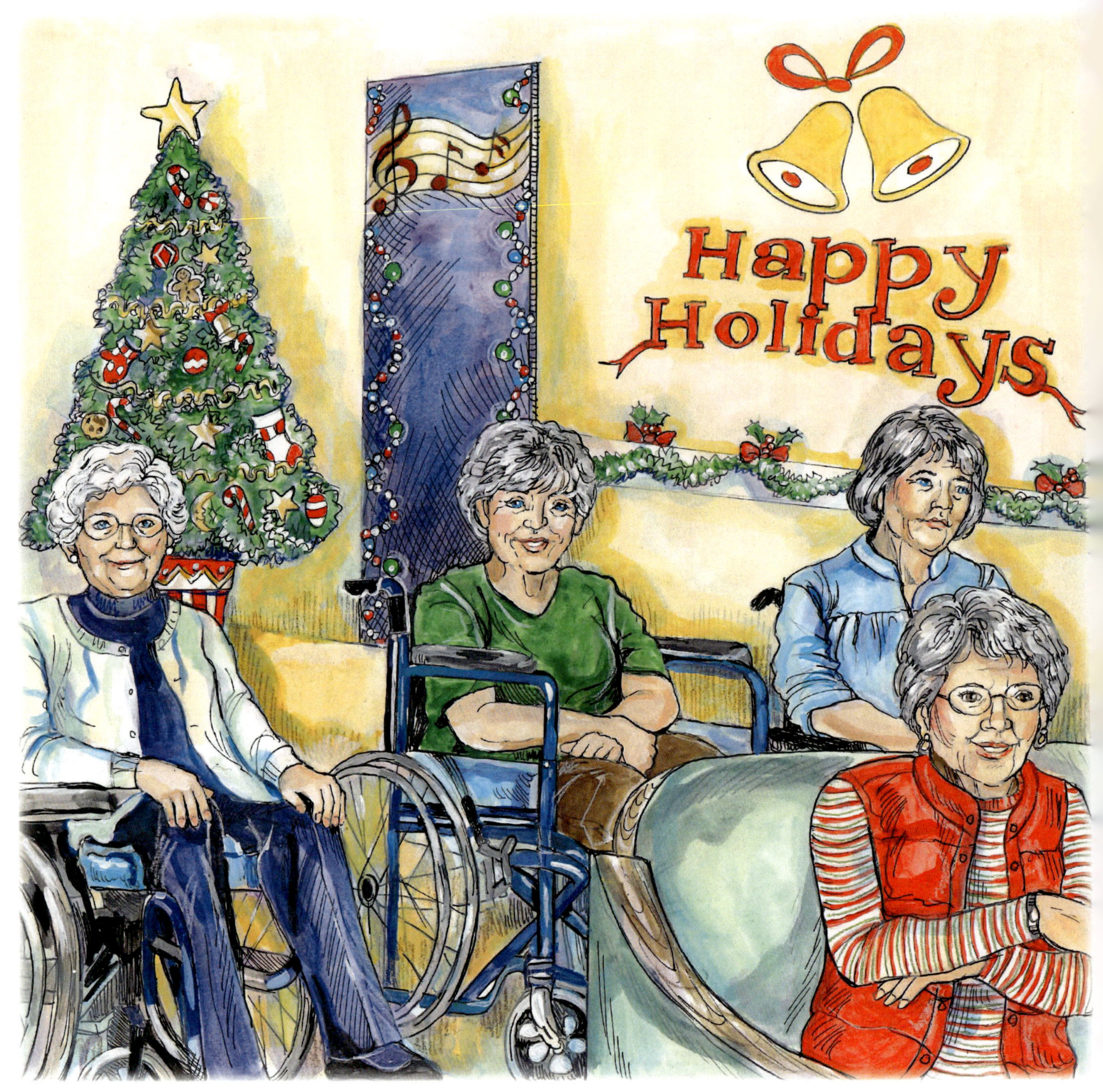

Great Grandma gathered with others for music, but no one was moving to the beat.

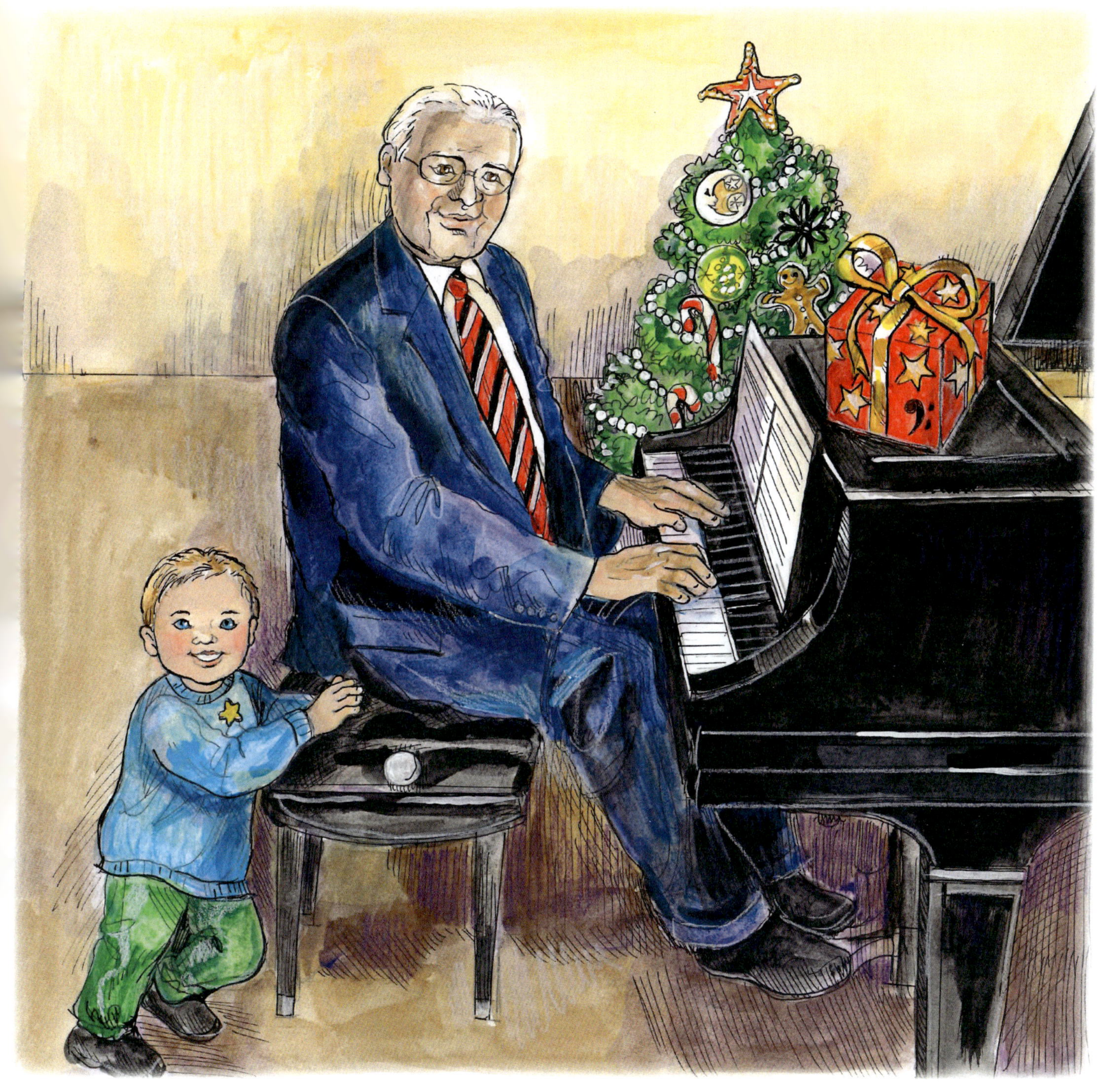

No one, that is, except Law. He always danced while Dave played. Since Law could barely stand, he hung onto the piano bench, bouncing and giggling.

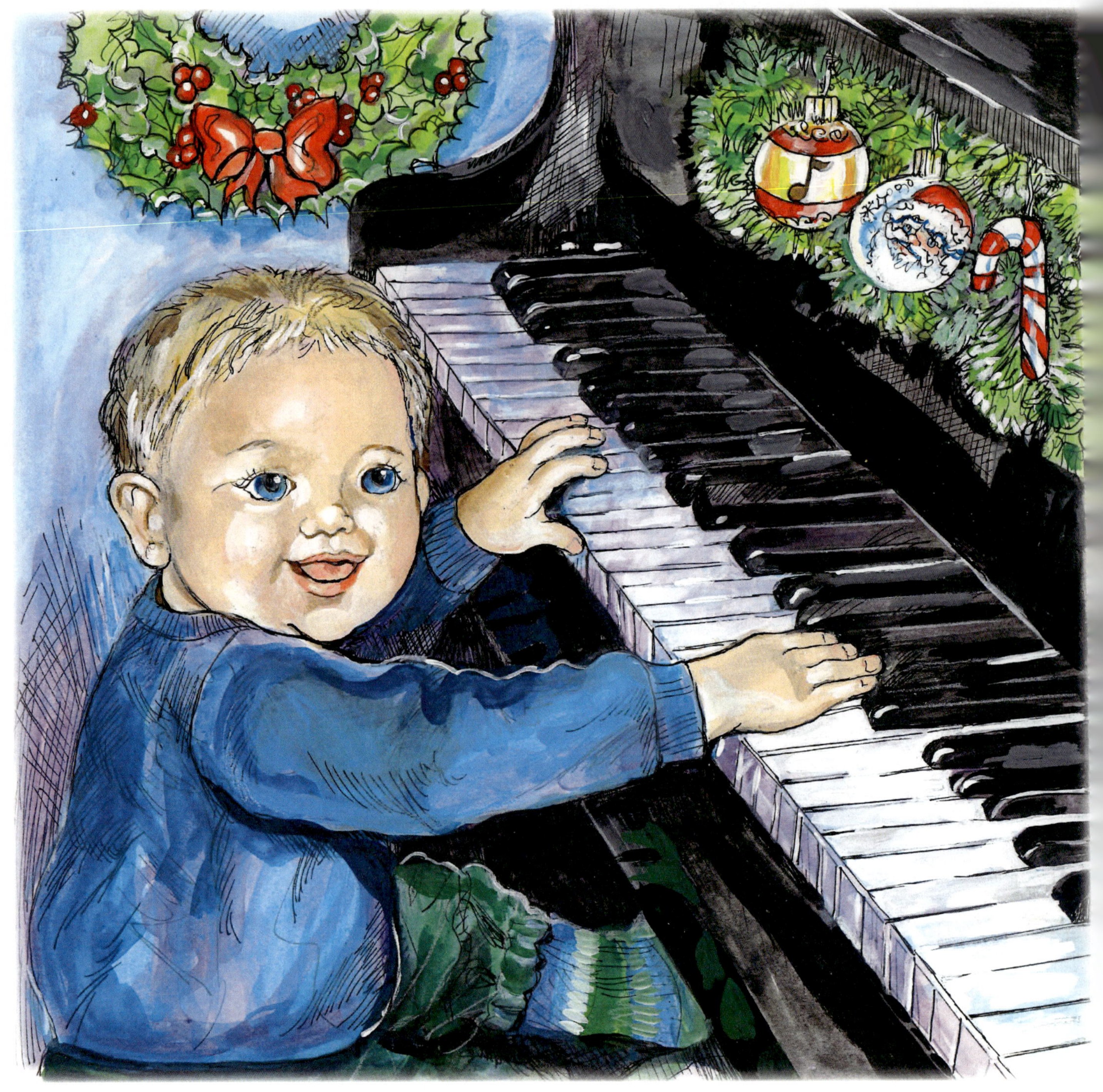

Sometimes Dave even let Law tinkle those piano keys. When the residents watched Law, they remembered their own children and applauded Law trying to play.

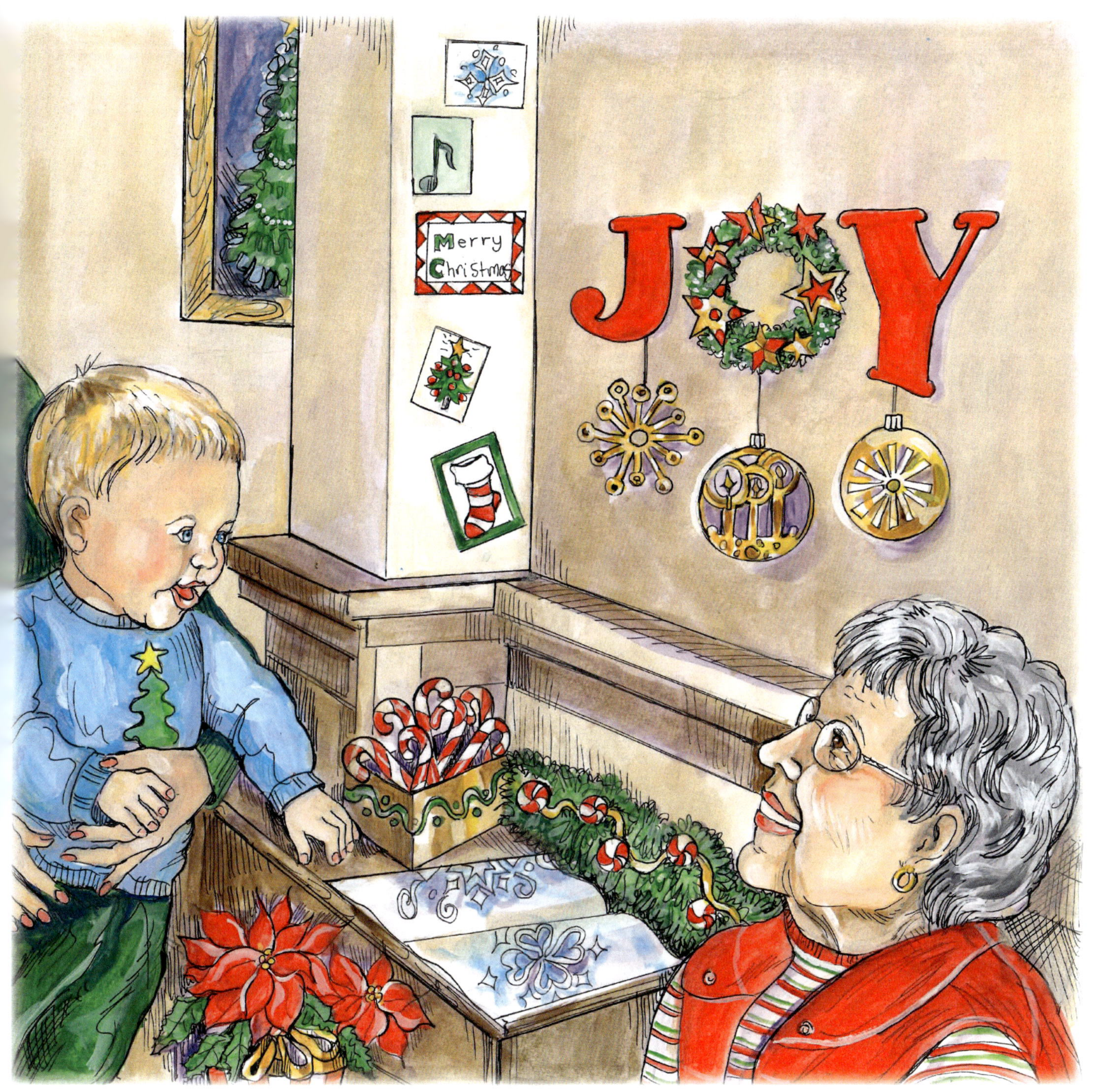

Great Grandma loved Law's weekly visits.

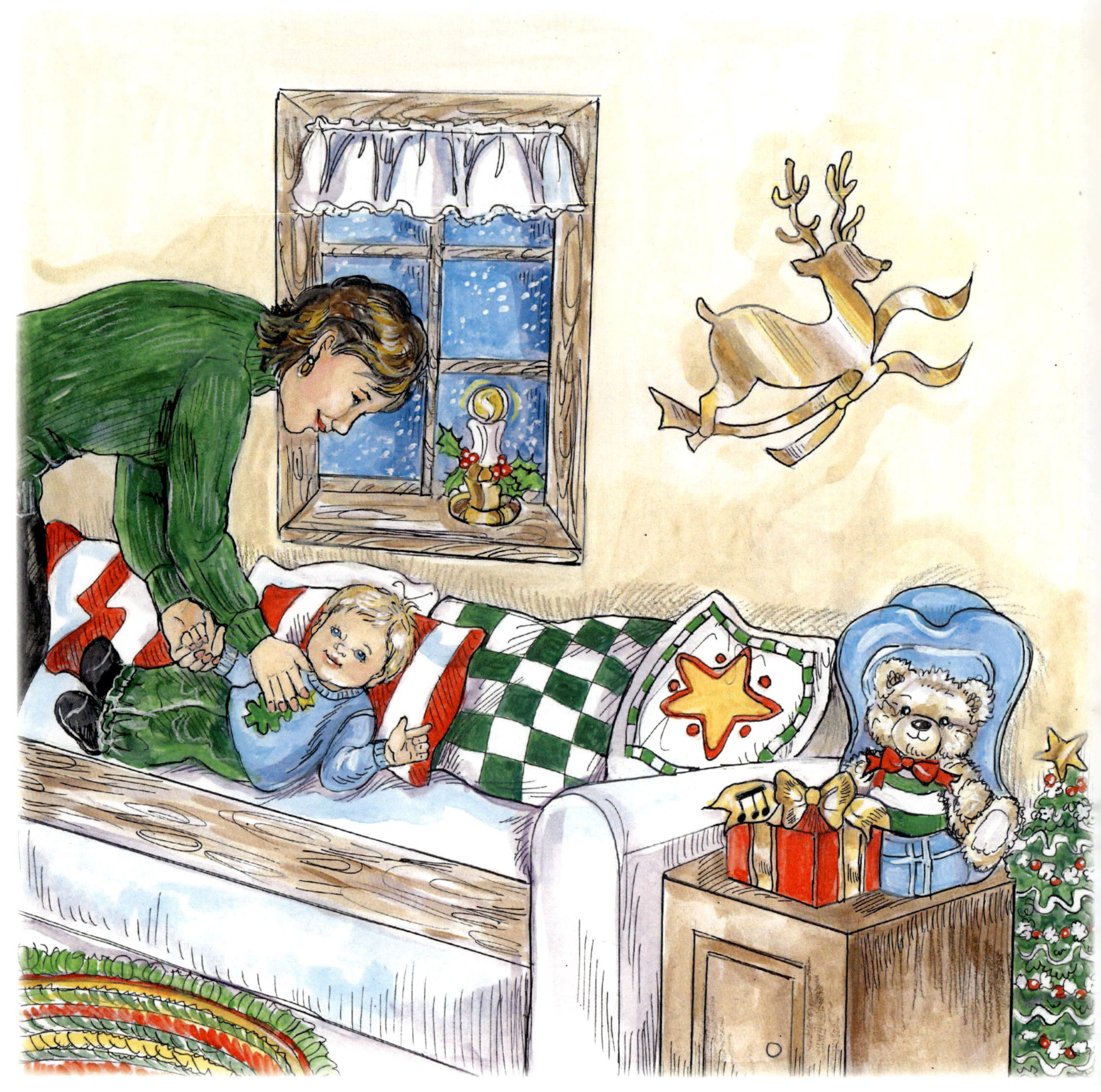

One day MiMi decided to liven up music hour by picking up Law and starting to dance.

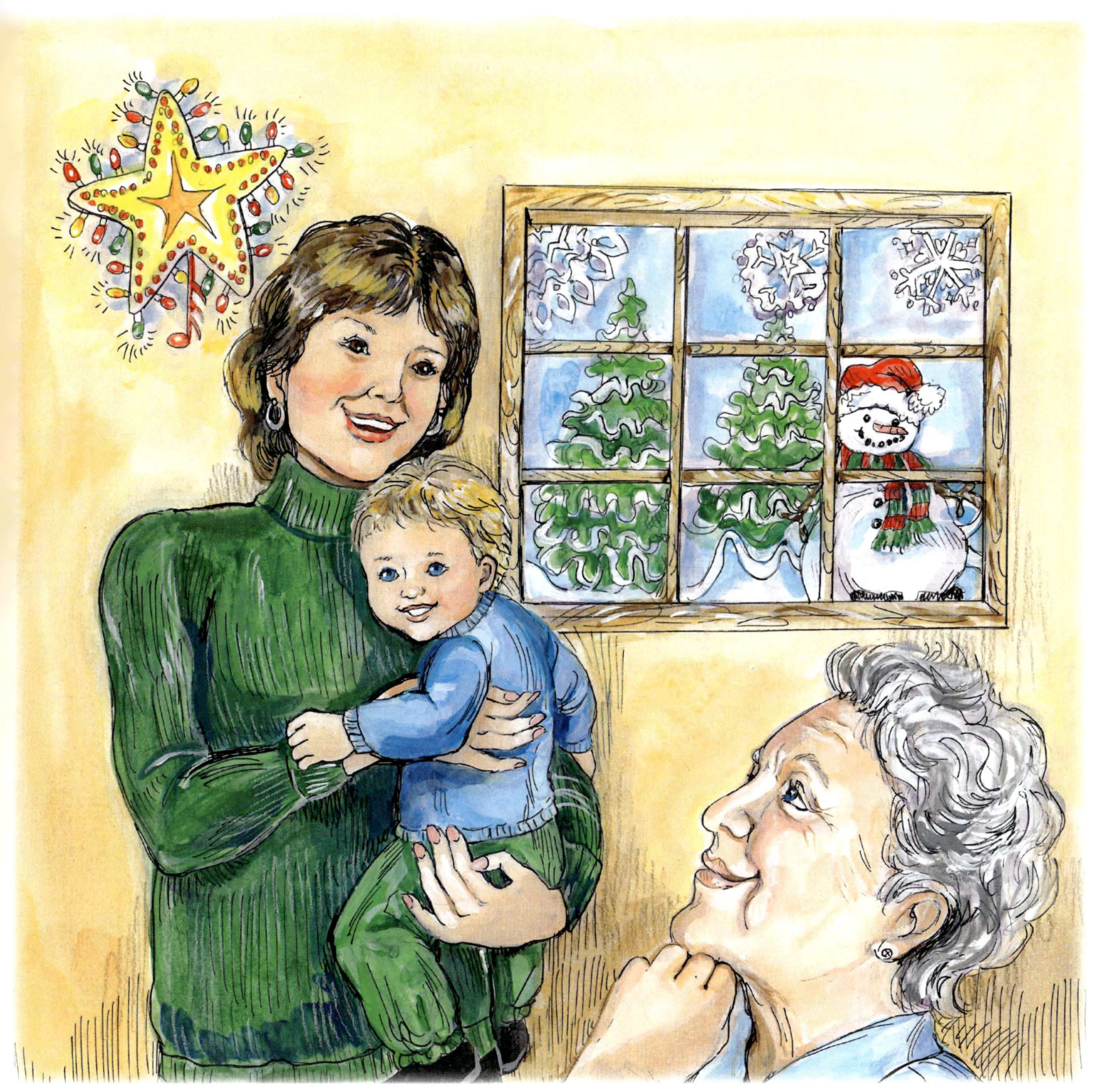

She waltzed and she tangoed around the room with Law on her hip.

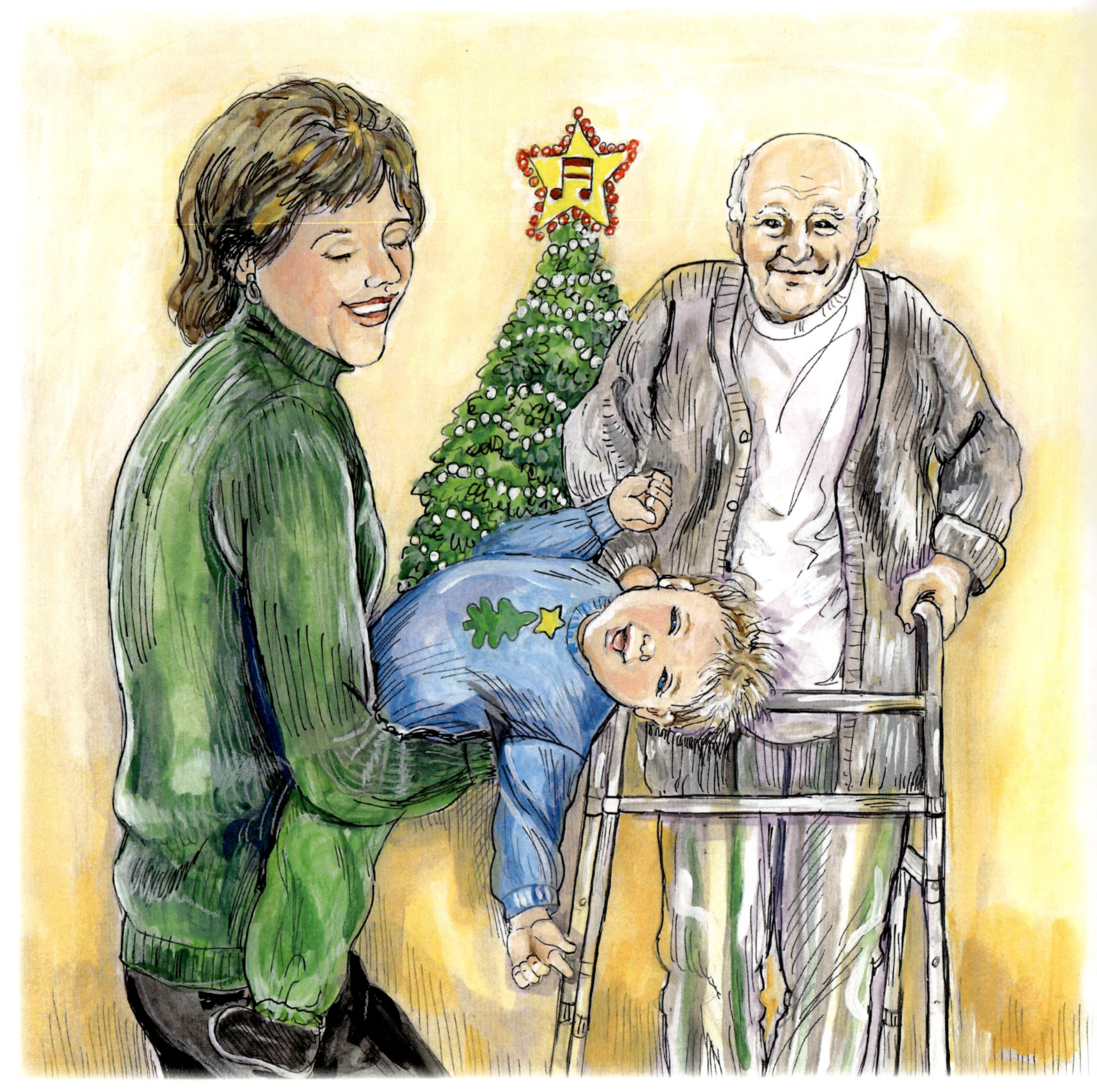

Each resident showed delight when MiMi and Law would pause for a dip.

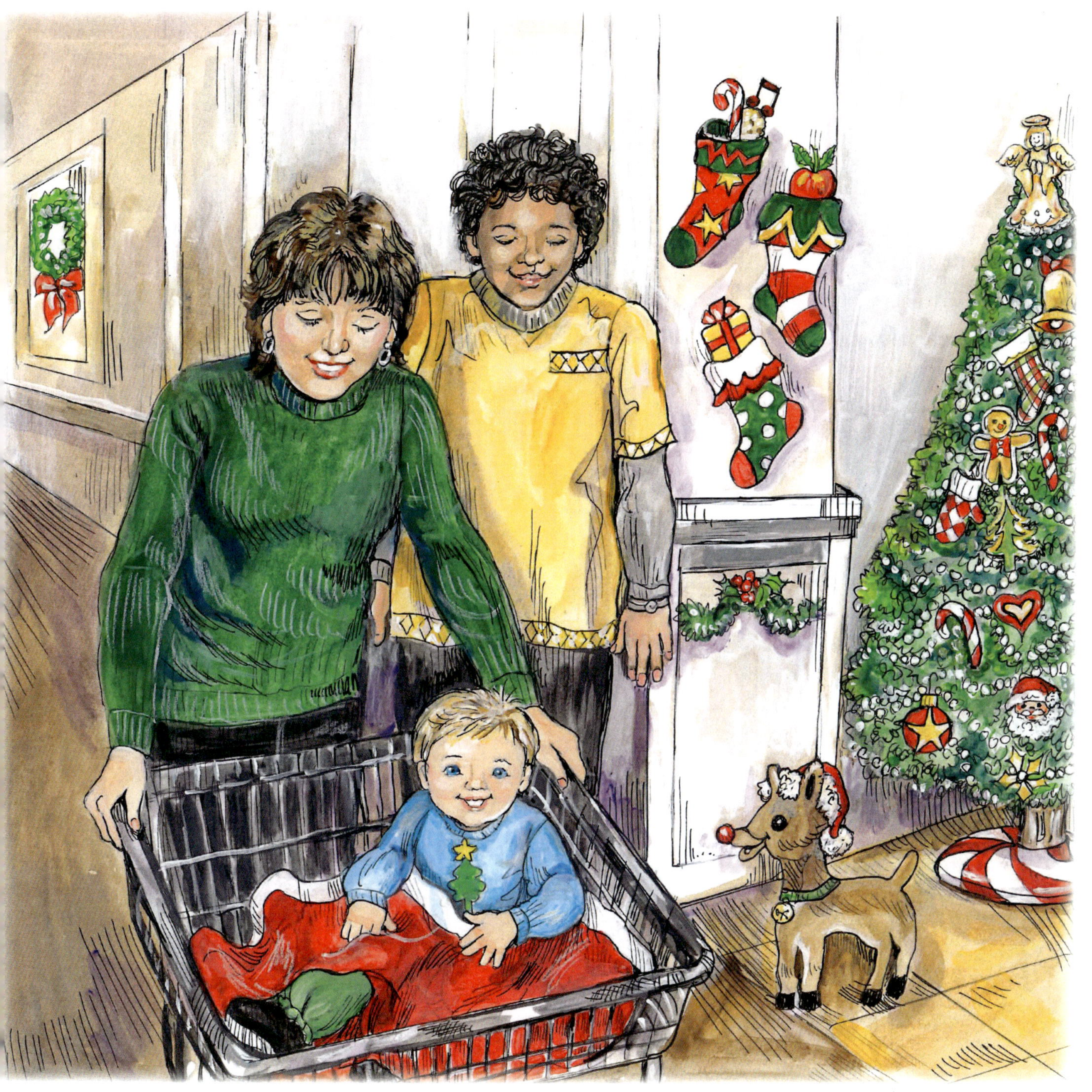

When MiMi's arms grew tired, the staff brought out a laundry cart so she could move easily as she continued to dance with Law.

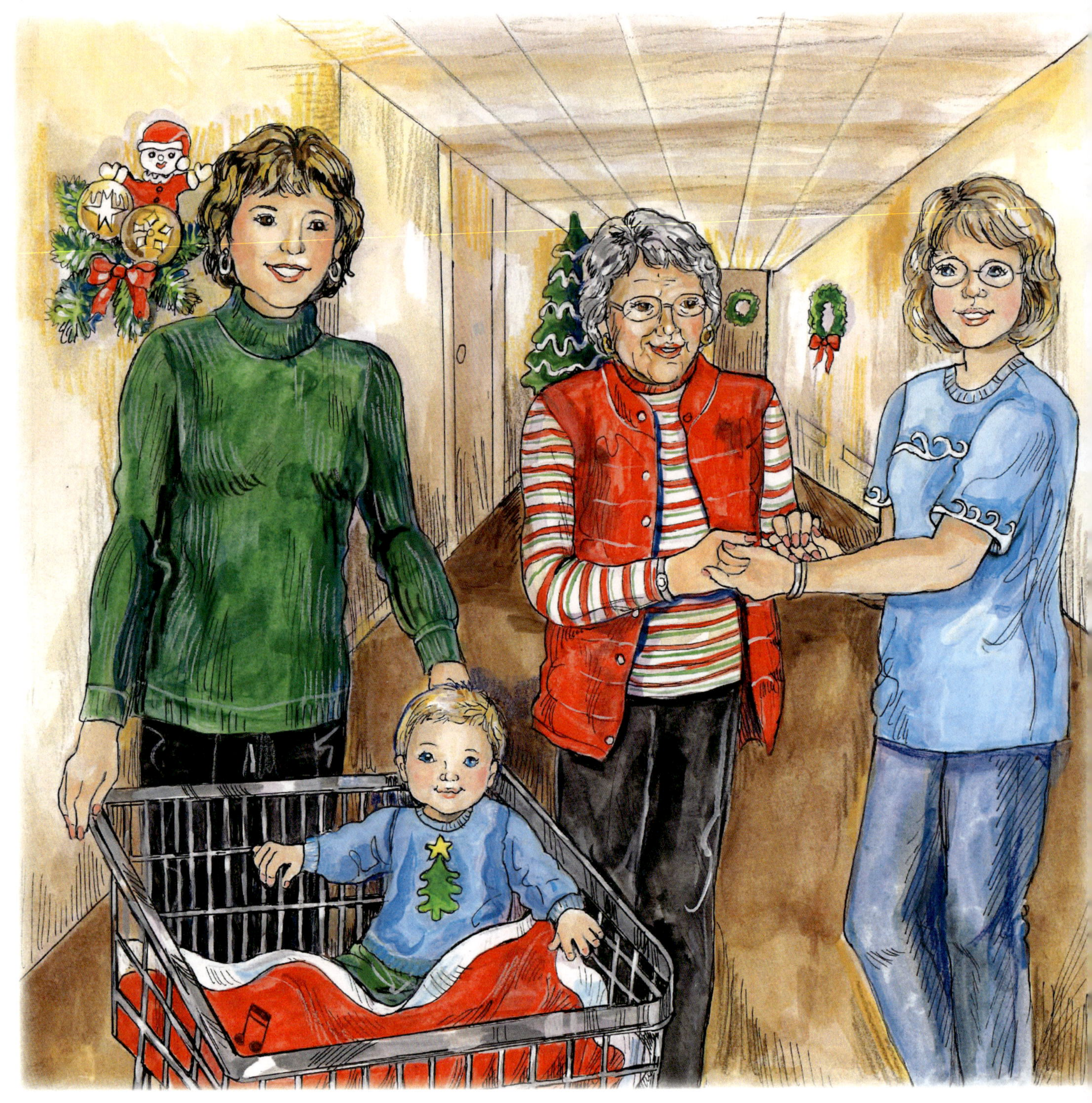

Law grooved in the basket, waving his arms and moving to the beat.

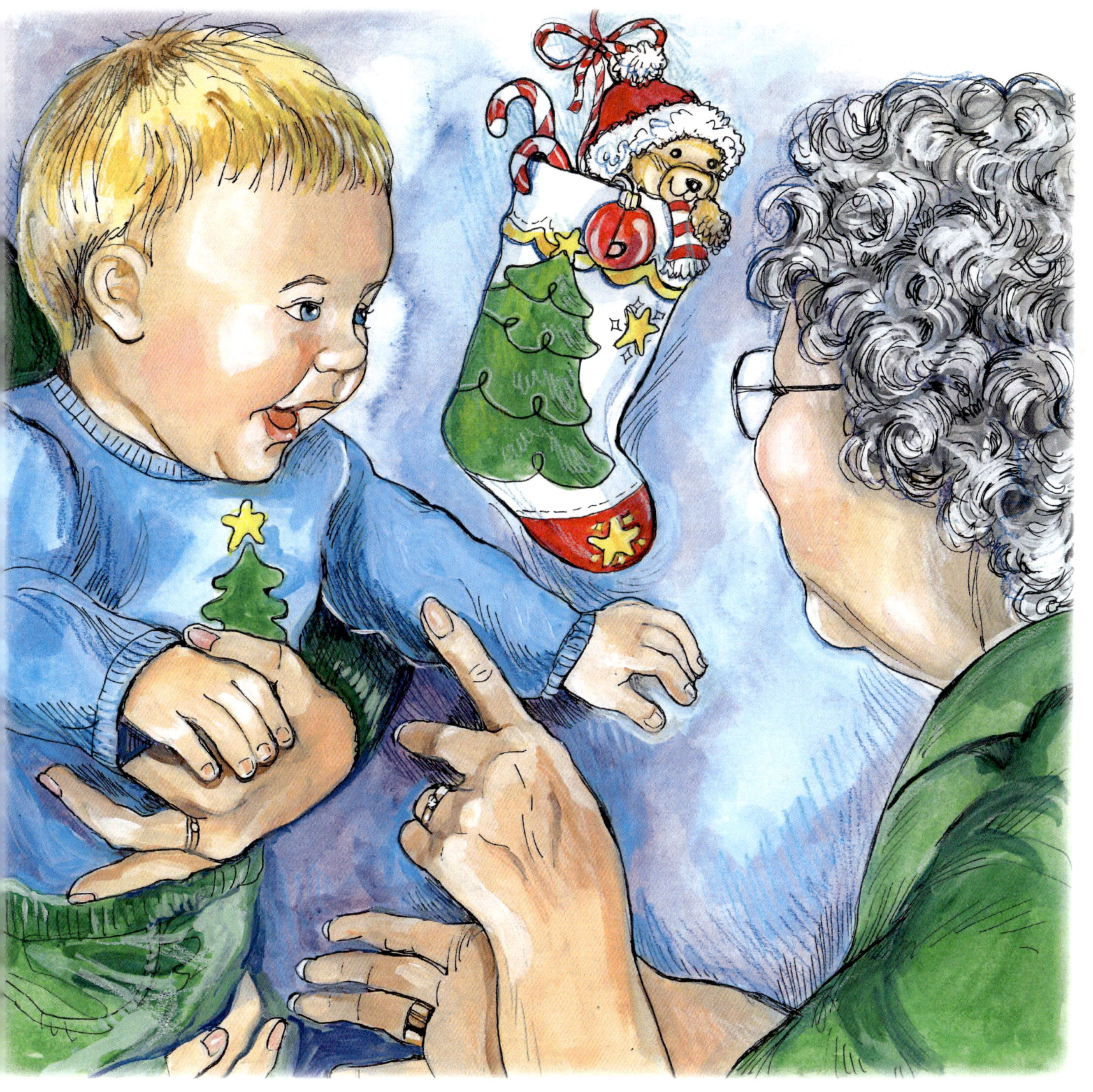

MiMi made sure each resident had a chance to “dance” with Law. Law would look into their eyes and smile as he passed by.

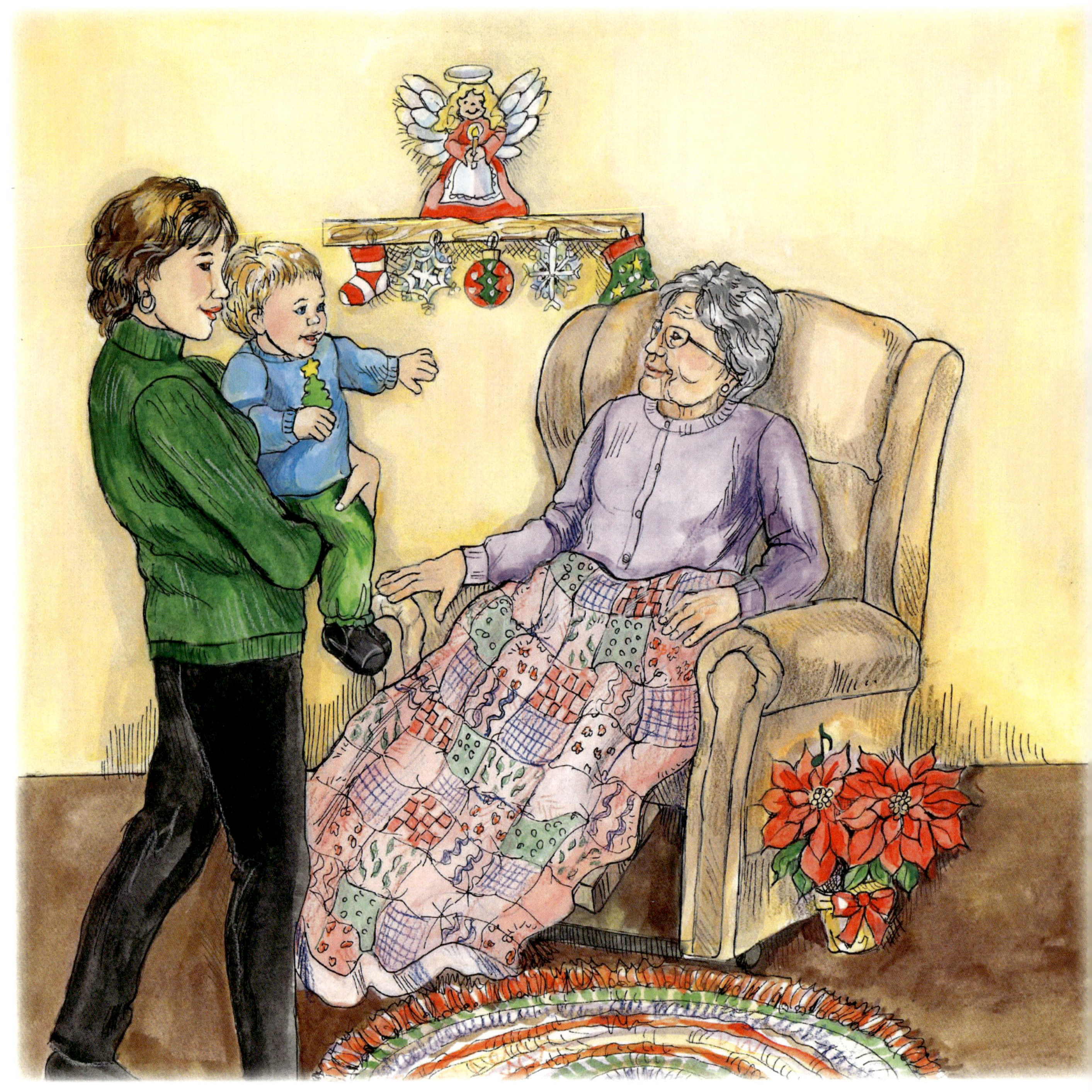

Some laughed while others had tears in their eyes as they thought of their pasts. Law kept moving to the beat.

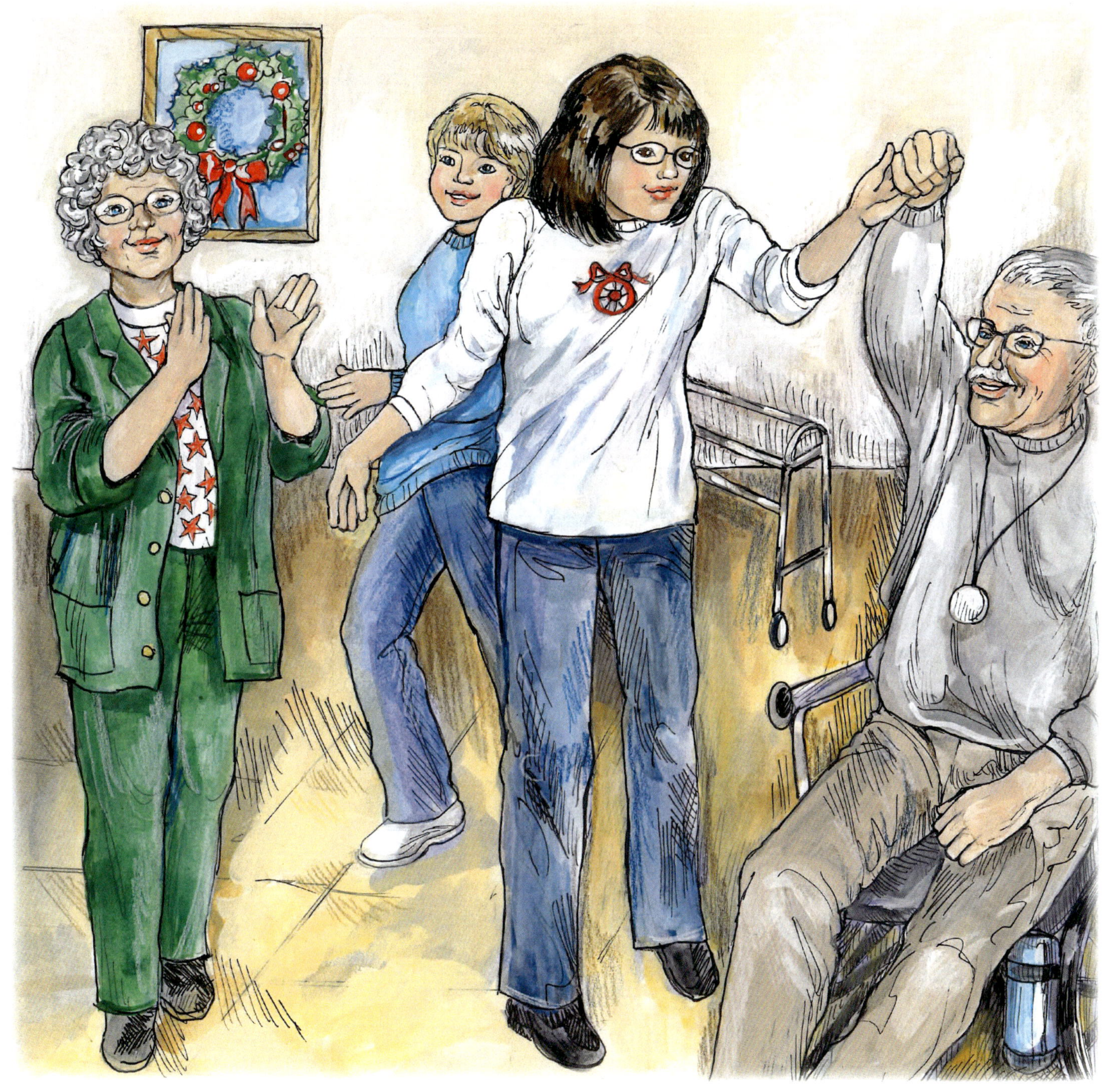

Pat Peters joined in. Evaline never stopped—she was a real dancing machine!

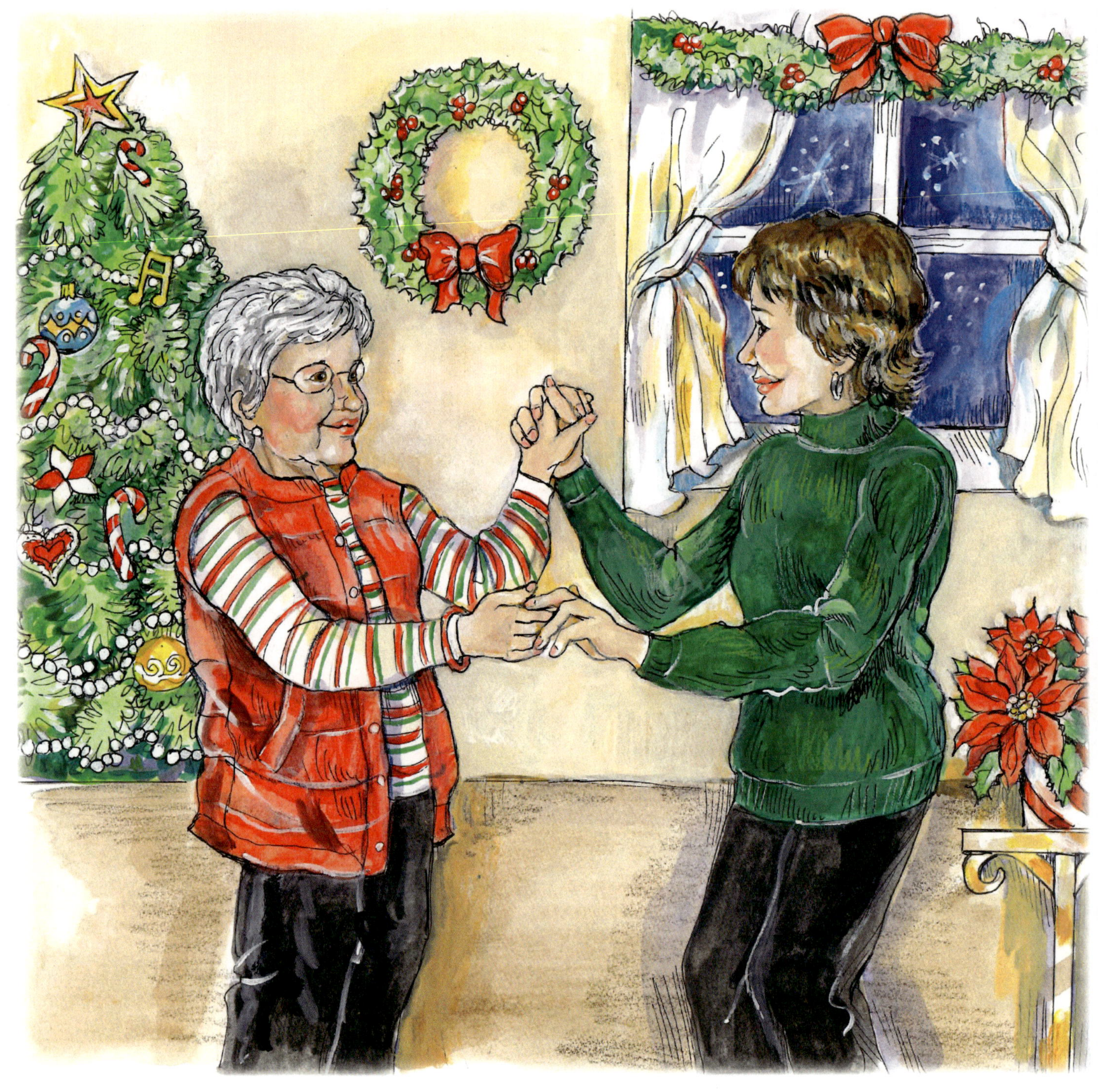

The whole staff was thrilled when Great Grandma put her walker aside and danced with MiMi.

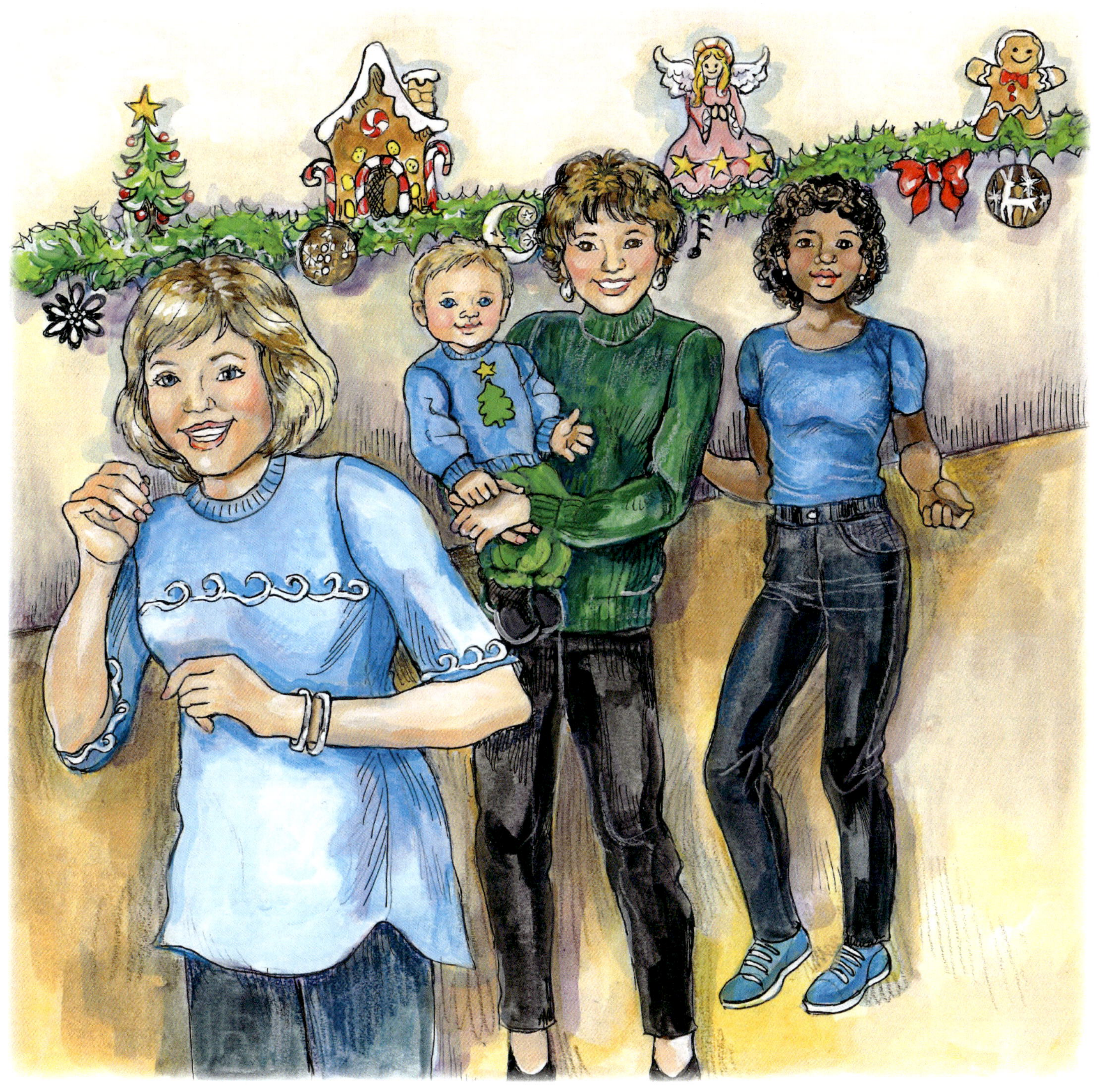

Later, a conga line was formed. Soon the staff, Law and MiMi were swaying down the hall.

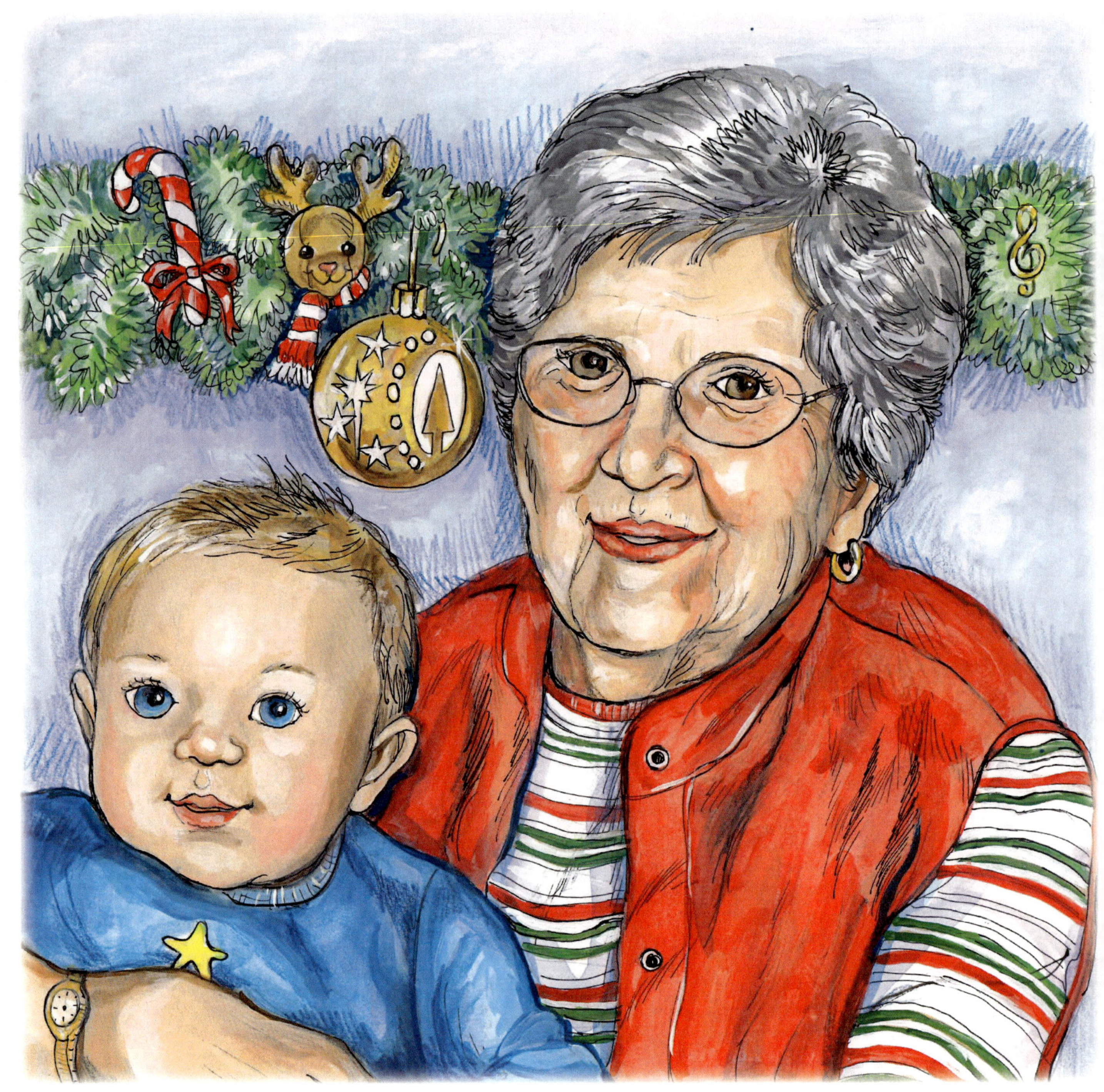

Knowing her great grandson had helped to brighten music time for the residents gave Great Grandma pride and joy.

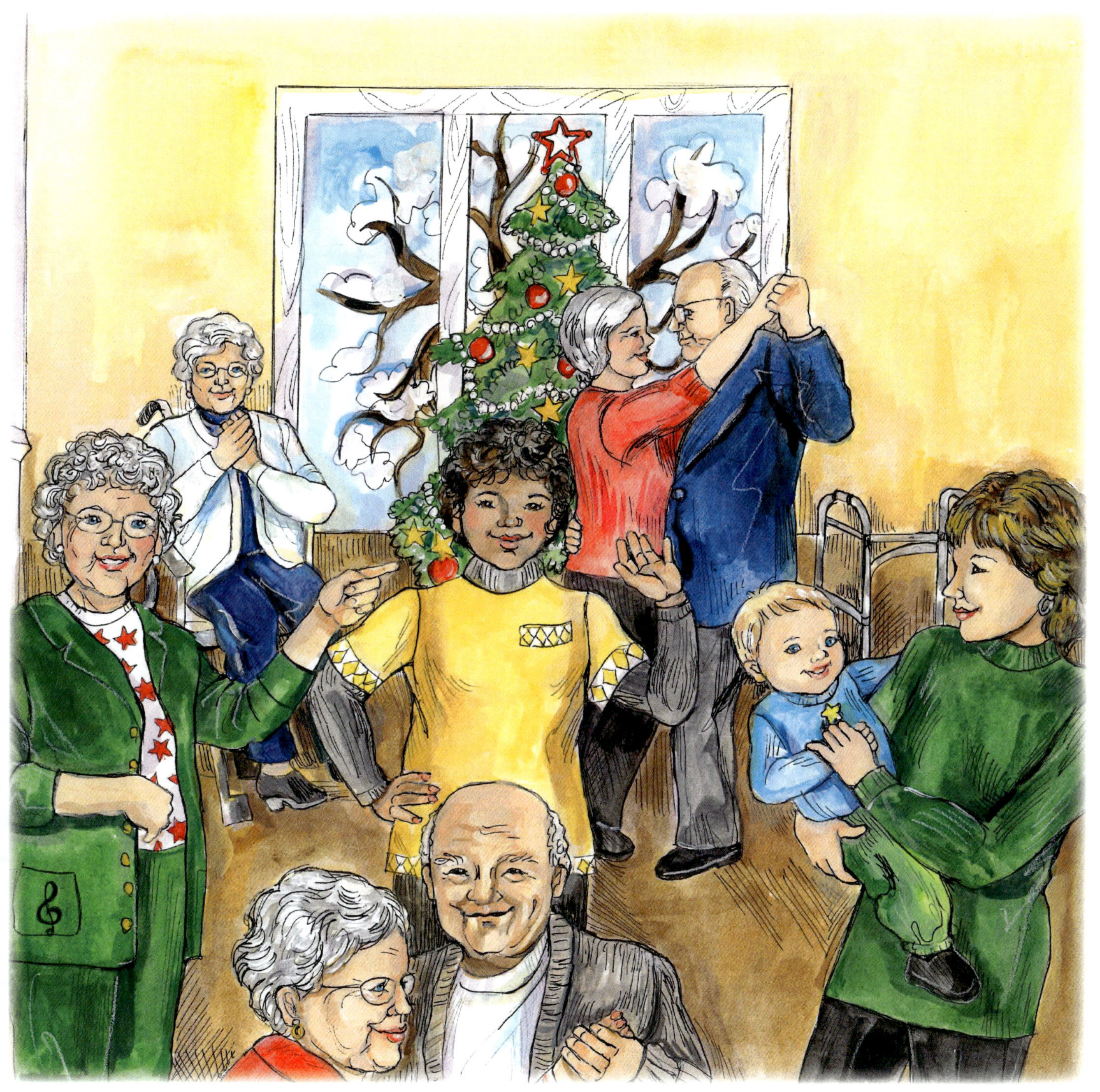

These musical Wednesdays were days when the elderly enjoyed fun and motion.

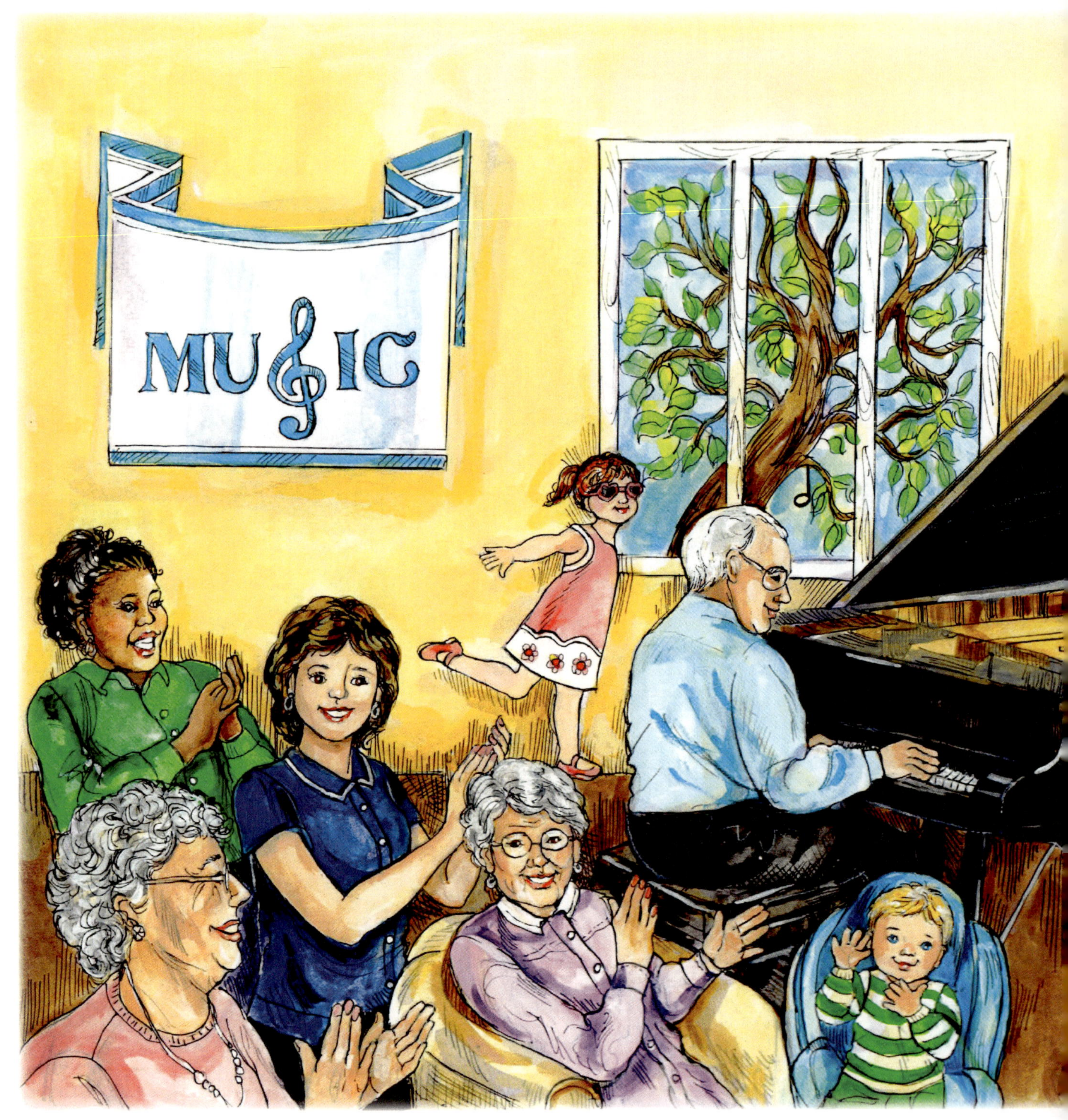

As time moved on and the weekly music continued …

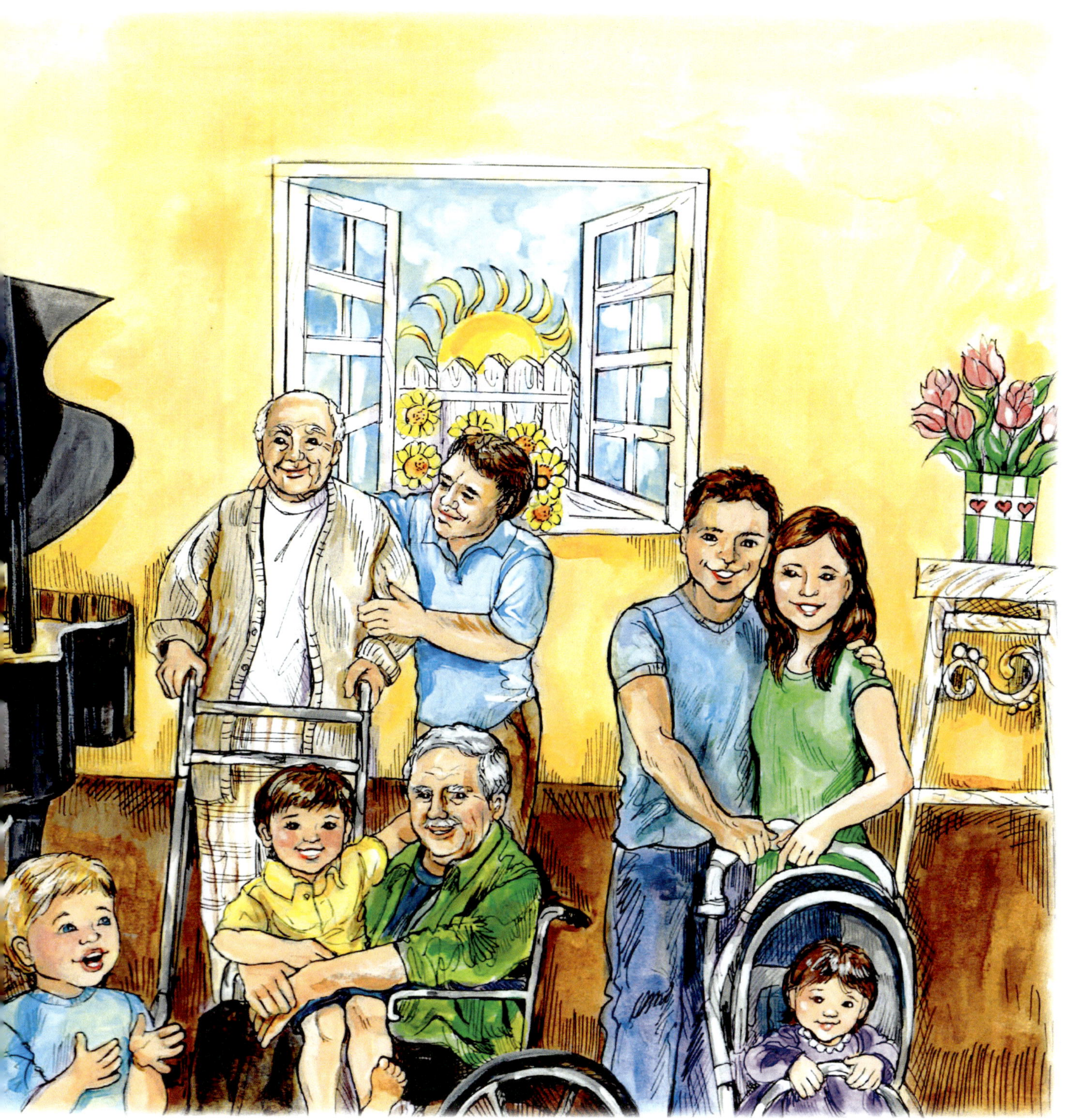

more families joined in to share dance, fun and song.

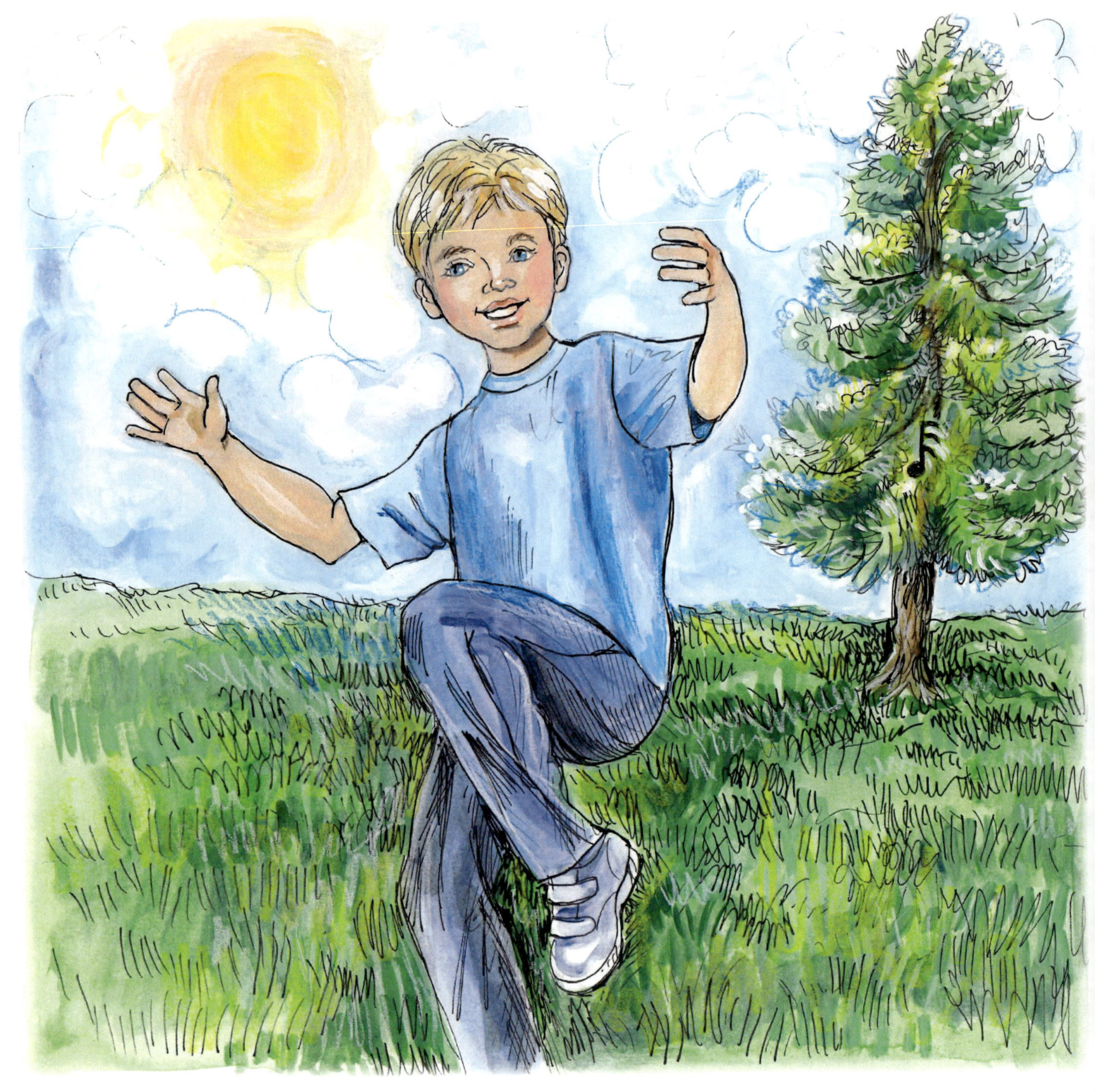

Eight years have passed. Law sure has grown. His love for music still shows.

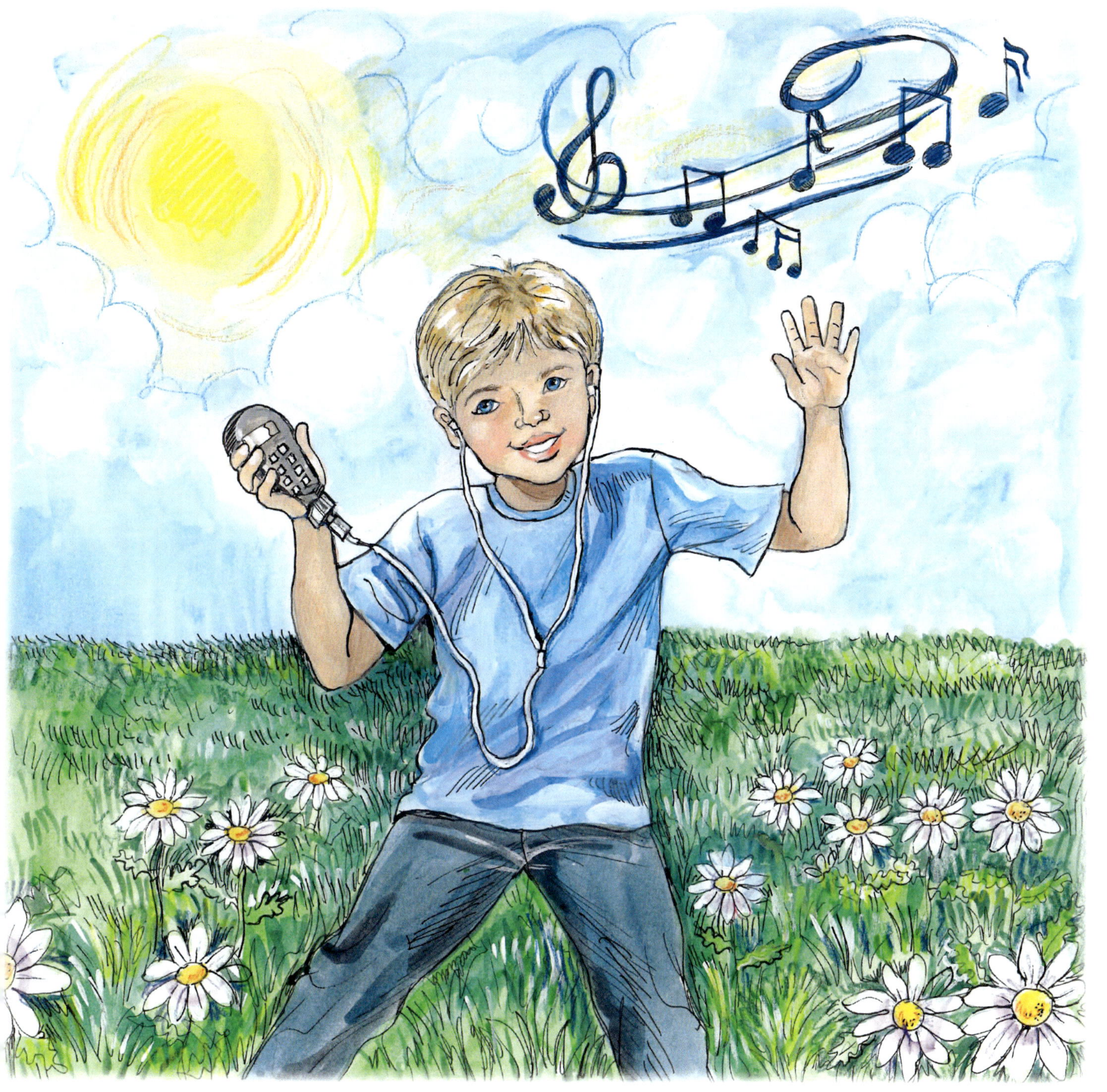

He moves to music: pop, rap, rock and roll…
We think Great Grandma's spirit is a part of his soul!

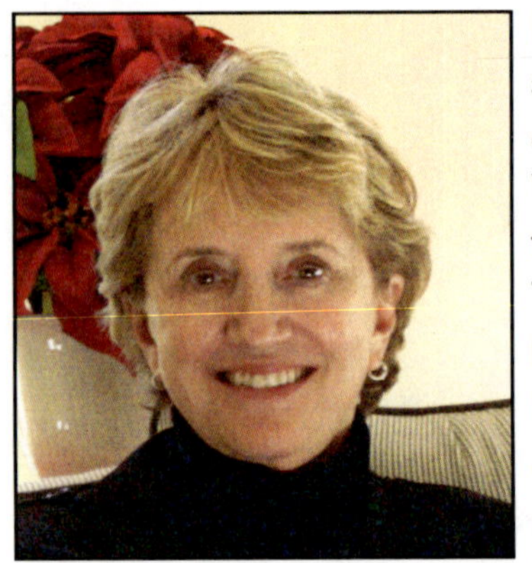

Rosalee Klopf Tithof is now enjoying her hobby of writing children's stories after retiring from her rewarding years as a secondary education teacher. She earned her bachelor's degree at Saginaw Valley State University and later studied in Mexico City. She taught school for a year in a U.S. State Department School in Torreon, Mexico, a year that her whole family agreed was one of the best of their lives. She finished her career teaching in Chesaning, Michigan. Her first book, *My Michigan Summer,* was published as an ebook and republished as a paperback book early in 2017 on Amazon. Her second book, *Remembering Pop Pop*, is also available on Amazon along with *Dancing with Great Grandma*. Each of the last two books highlights a grandchild so there is need for two more books to be written as Ms. Tithof has four loving grandkids. Rose spends her winters in the Southwest and summers in Michigan.

Carilyn Teichman is from Owosso, Michigan. In 1980 she graduated from The Art Institute of Pittsburgh with a degree in Fashion Illustration. She has over 30 years of experience as a professional illustrator which includes working as an illustrator in an advertising department and as an artist at a collectibles company. She worked at a sportswear company where her designs were embroidered on clothing and as an artist for a silkscreen printer.

Carilyn has illustrated paper doll sets for Pratt & Austin and paper dolls for magazines such as *Contemporary Doll Collector Magazine and Miniature Collector.* She also illustrated the children's book, *Remembering Pop Pop.*

When I visited my mother during her time in the assisted living home, I realized that joining in the games and fun made her stay and my visits more enjoyable. I will never regret the conversations we had during those visits, as I learned things about her life I never would have known.

Come Visit Me

Come visit me, won't you please?
Although I am ailing, not moving very well,
I'd love to reminisce with you—great stories I can tell!

These stories I'll share if you'll listen to me.
A caring nurse and a mother whose kids grew so fast.
Now a keeper of memories of a life so quickly passed.

Just come and visit so you will know
What life was like so long ago.
Fond recollections you will hear
Of all the moments I hold dear.

Lawrence Danek and Dave Rusz reunited for more music. August 2017

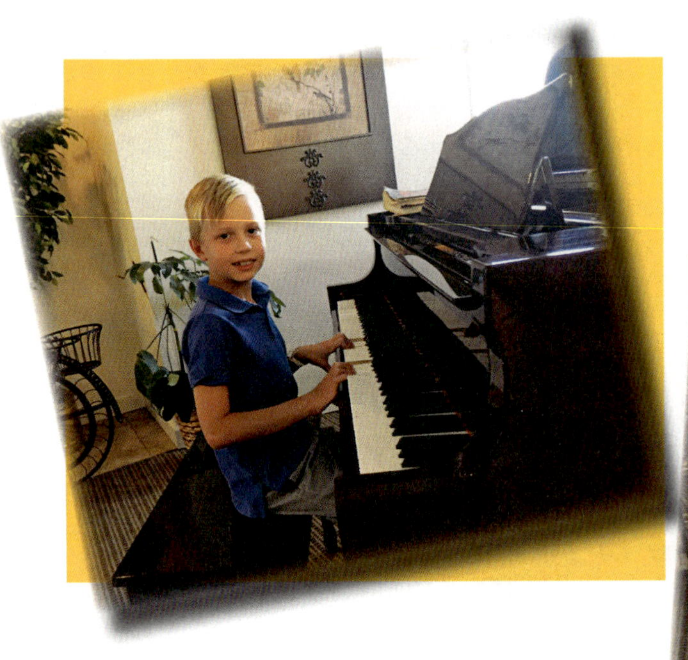

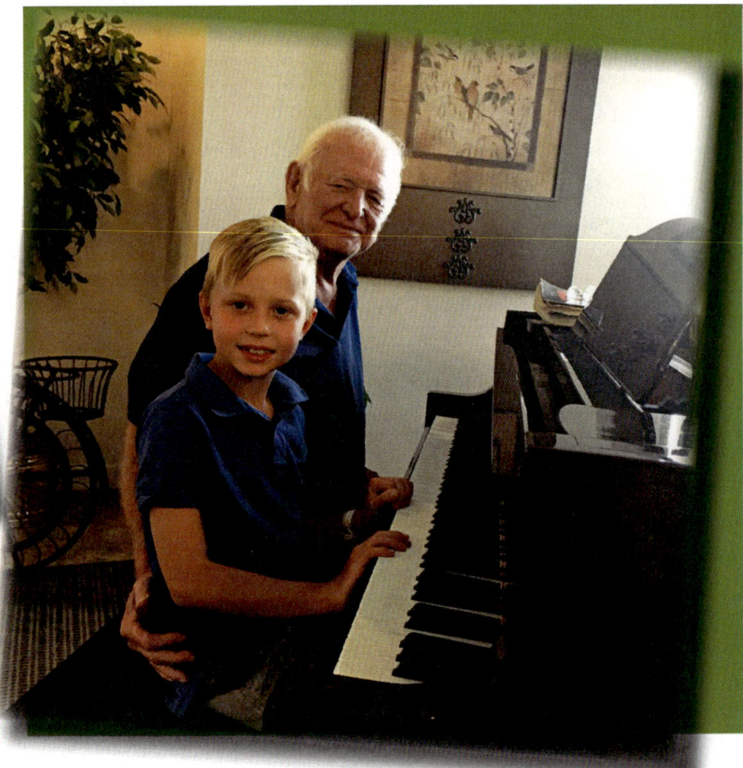

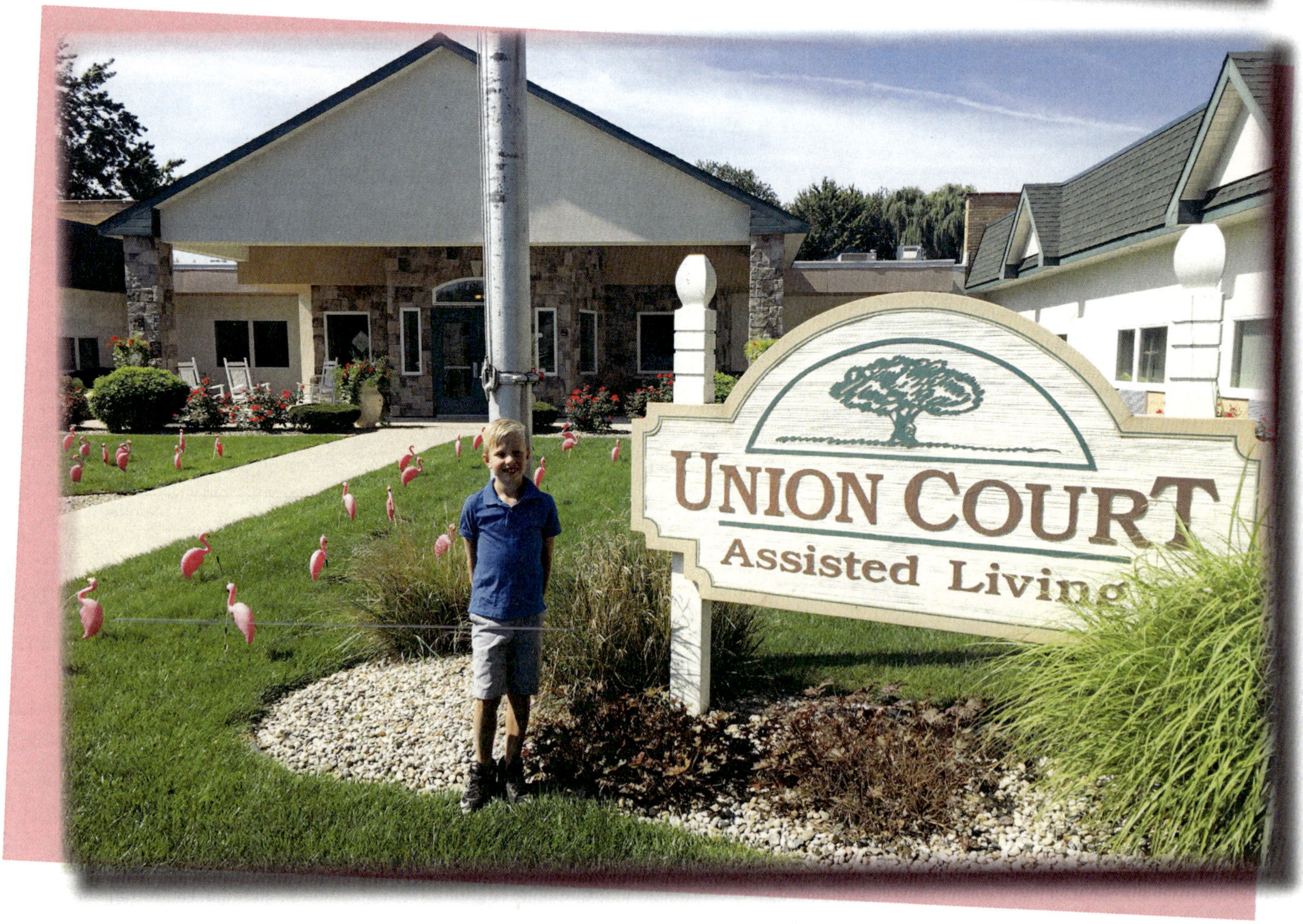